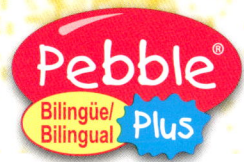

¿QUÉ HAY EN MiPlato?

WHAT'S ON MyPlate?

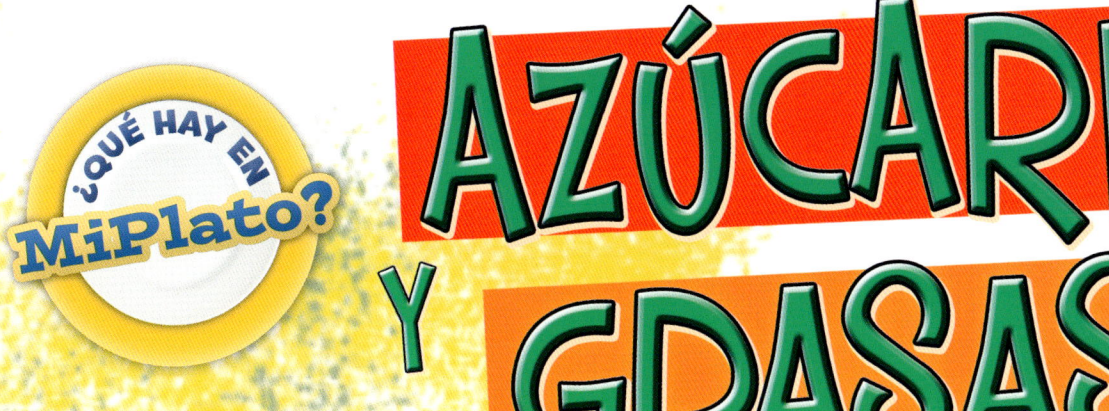

AZÚCARES Y GRASAS
SUGARS AND FATS

por/by Mari Schuh

Editora consultora/Consulting Editor:
Gail Saunders-Smith, PhD

Consultora/Consultant: Barbara J. Rolls, PhD
Guthrie Chair en Nutrición/Guthrie Chair in Nutrition
Pennsylvania State University
University Park, Pennsylvania

CAPSTONE PRESS
a capstone imprint

Pebble Plus is published by Capstone Press,
1710 Roe Crest Drive, North Mankato, Minnesota 56003
www.capstonepub.com

Copyright © 2013 by Capstone Press, a Capstone imprint. All rights reserved. No part of this publication may be reproduced in whole or in part, or stored in a retrieval system, or transmitted in any form or by any means, electronic, mechanical, photocopying, recording, or otherwise, without written permission of the publisher.

Library of Congress Cataloging-in-Publication Data
Schuh, Mari C., 1975–
 [Sugars and fats.]
 Azúcares y grasas = Sugars and fats / por Mari Schuh.
    pages cm.—(Pebble Plus bilingüe. ¿Qué hay en miplato? = Pebble Plus bilingual. What's on myplate?)
 Audience: Grades K to 3.
 Includes index.
 ISBN 978-1-62065-946-5 (library binding)
 ISBN 978-1-4765-1752-0 (ebook PDF)
 1. Sugars in human nutrition—Juvenile literature. 2. Oils and fats—Juvenile literature. 3. Confectionery—Juvenile literature. 4. Nutrition—Juvenile literature. I. Schuh, Mari C., 1975– Sugars and fats II. Schuh, Mari C., 1975– Sugars and fats. Spanish. III. Title. IV. Title: Sugars and fats.
 TX553.S8S3818 2013
 612.3'96—dc23   2012022649

Summary: Simple text and photos describe USDA's MyPlate tool and healthy sugar and fat choices for children—in both English and Spanish

Editorial Credits
Jeni Wittrock, editor; Strictly Spanish, translation services; Gene Bentdahl, designer; Eric Manske, bilingual book designer; Svetlana Zhurkin, media researcher; Jennifer Walker, production specialist; Sarah Schuette, photo stylist; Marcy Morin, studio scheduler

Photo Credits
All photos by Capstone Studio/Karon Dubke except:
Shutterstock: Anna Subbotina, back cover, Mark Stout Photography, cover; USDA, cover (inset), 5

The author dedicates this book to Travis Rusche, who loves to get his head around health.

Information in this book supports the U.S. Department of Agriculture's MyPlate food guidance system found at www.choosemyplate.gov. Food amounts listed in this book are based on daily recommendations for children ages 4-8. The amounts listed in this book are appropriate for children who get less than 30 minutes a day of moderate physical activity, beyond normal daily activities. Children who are more physically active may be able to eat more while staying within calorie needs. The U.S. Department of Agriculture (USDA) does not endorse any products, services, or organizations.

Note to Parents and Teachers

The ¿Qué hay en MiPlato?/What's on MyPlate? series supports national science standards related to health and nutrition. This book describes and illustrates the USDA's recommendations on sugars and fats. The images support early readers in understanding the text. The repetition of words and phrases helps early readers learn new words. This book also introduces early readers to subject-specific vocabulary words, which are defined in the Glossary section. Early readers may need assistance to read some words and to use the Table of Contents, Glossary, Internet Sites, and Index sections of the book.

Printed in China.
092012   006934LEOS13

Table of Contents

MyPlate 4
Sugars and Fats 6
Eat Smart 12
Making Healthy Choices 20
Glossary 22
Internet Sites 22
Index 24

Tabla de contenidos

MiPlato 4
Azúcares y grasas 6
Come inteligentemente 12
Cómo hacer selecciones saludables 21
Glosario 23
Sitios de Internet 23
Índice 24

MyPlate/ MiPlato

MyPlate is a tool that helps you eat healthful food. MyPlate reminds you to limit the added sugars and solid fats that you eat.

MiPlato es una herramienta que te ayuda a comer alimentos saludables. MiPlato te hace recordar que tienes que limitar el azúcar agregada y las grasas sólidas que comes.

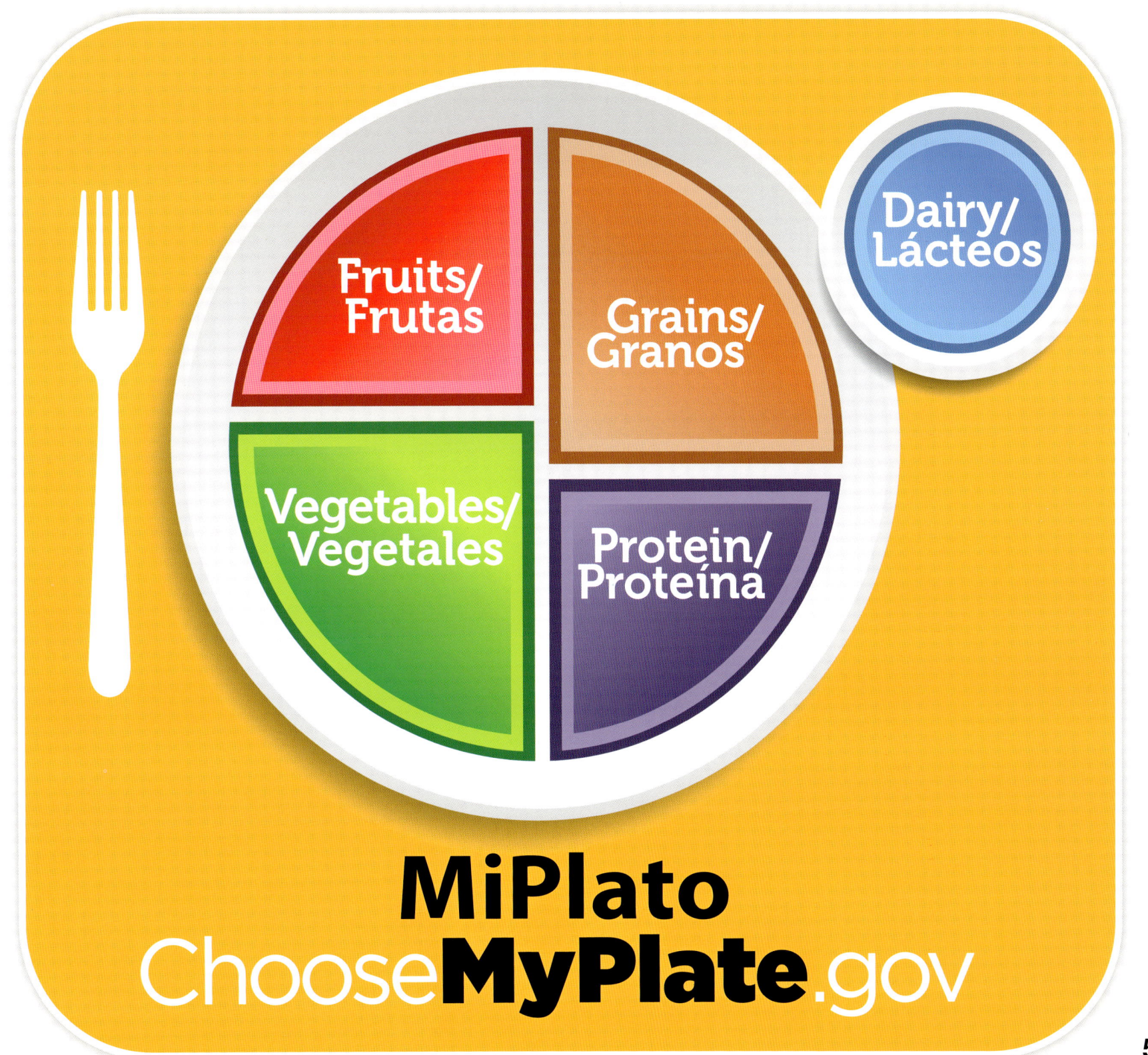

Sugars and Fats/ Azúcares y grasas

Sugar has very few nutrients. Some foods have natural sugars, such as fresh fruit. Avoid foods with added sugar.

El azúcar tiene muy pocos nutrientes. Algunos alimentos tienen azúcar natural, como la fruta fresca. Evita comer alimentos con azúcar agregada.

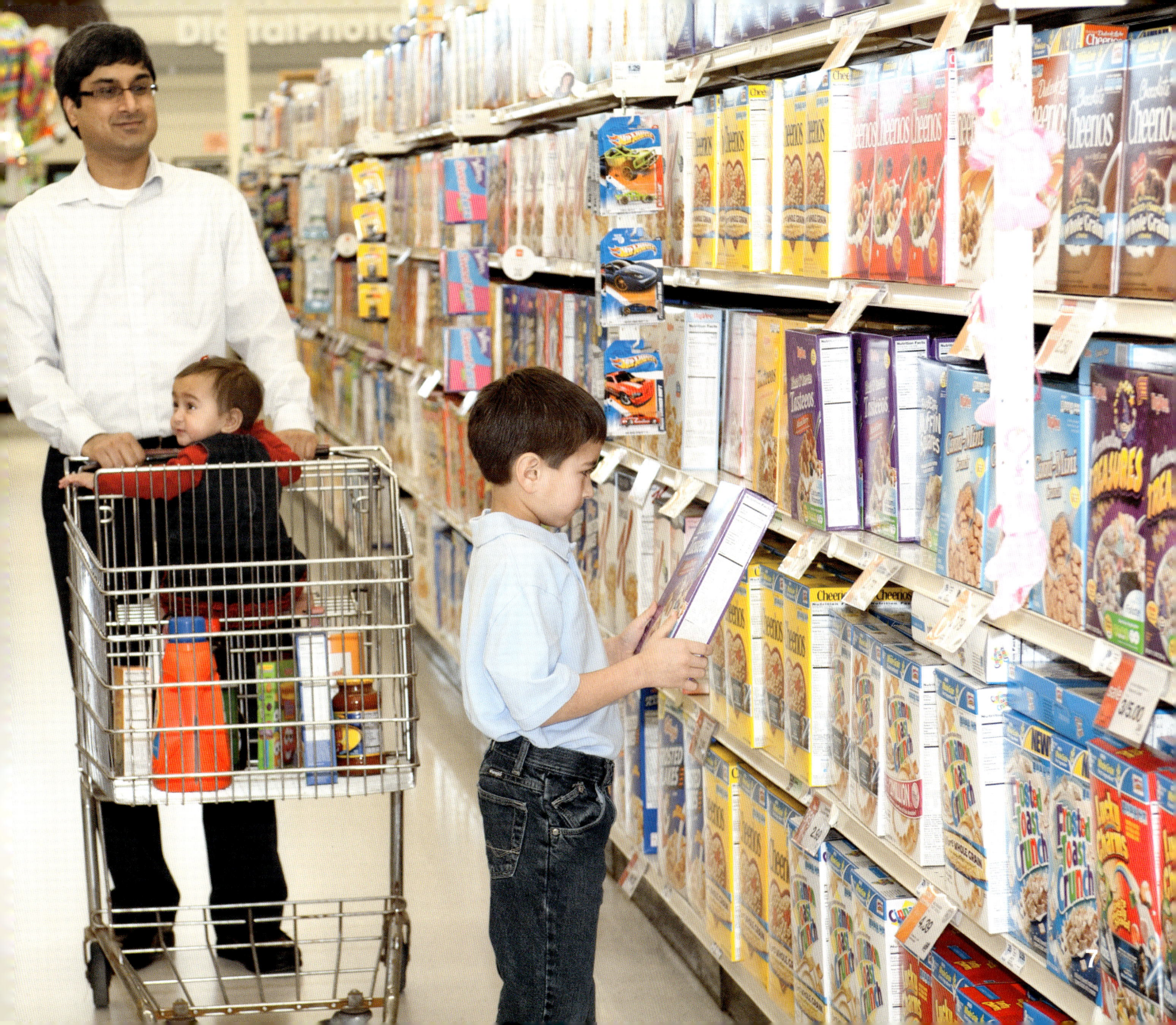

Everyone needs to eat some fat.

It has nutrients.

But some fats are better than others.

Eat fewer foods with solid fats, like french fries.

Todos necesitamos comer algo de grasa.

Tiene nutrientes.

Pero algunas grasas son mejores que otras.

Come menos alimentos con grasas sólidas, como las papas fritas.

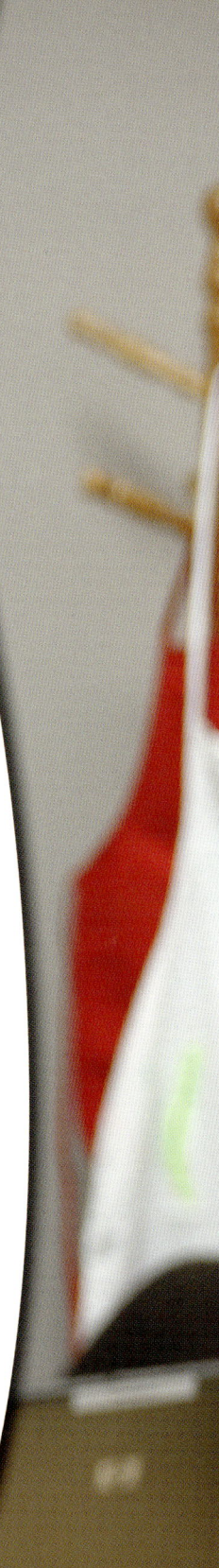

FAT FACTS
good
for you
Monounsaturated Fat
Polyunsaturated Fat
not-so-bad
for you
not-so-good
for you
Trans Fat
bad
for you

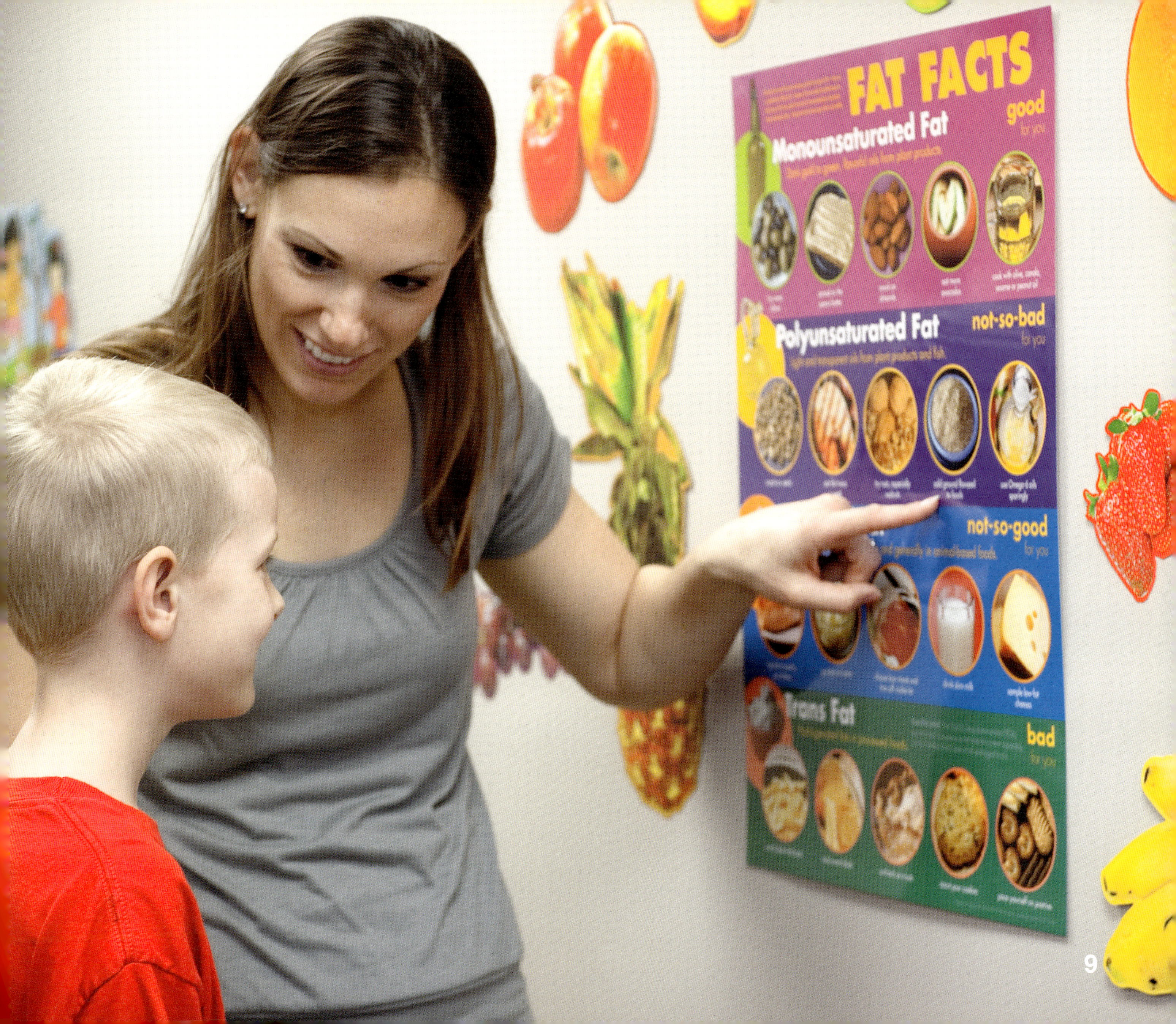

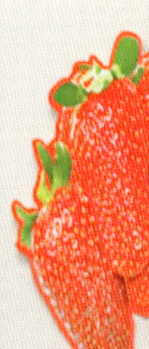

To grow healthy and strong,
limit your added sugars
and solid fats every day.
Eat sweets only as a special treat.

Para crecer saludable y fuerte,
limita el azúcar agregada y las
grasas sólidas todos los días.
Come dulces solo como una golosina especial.

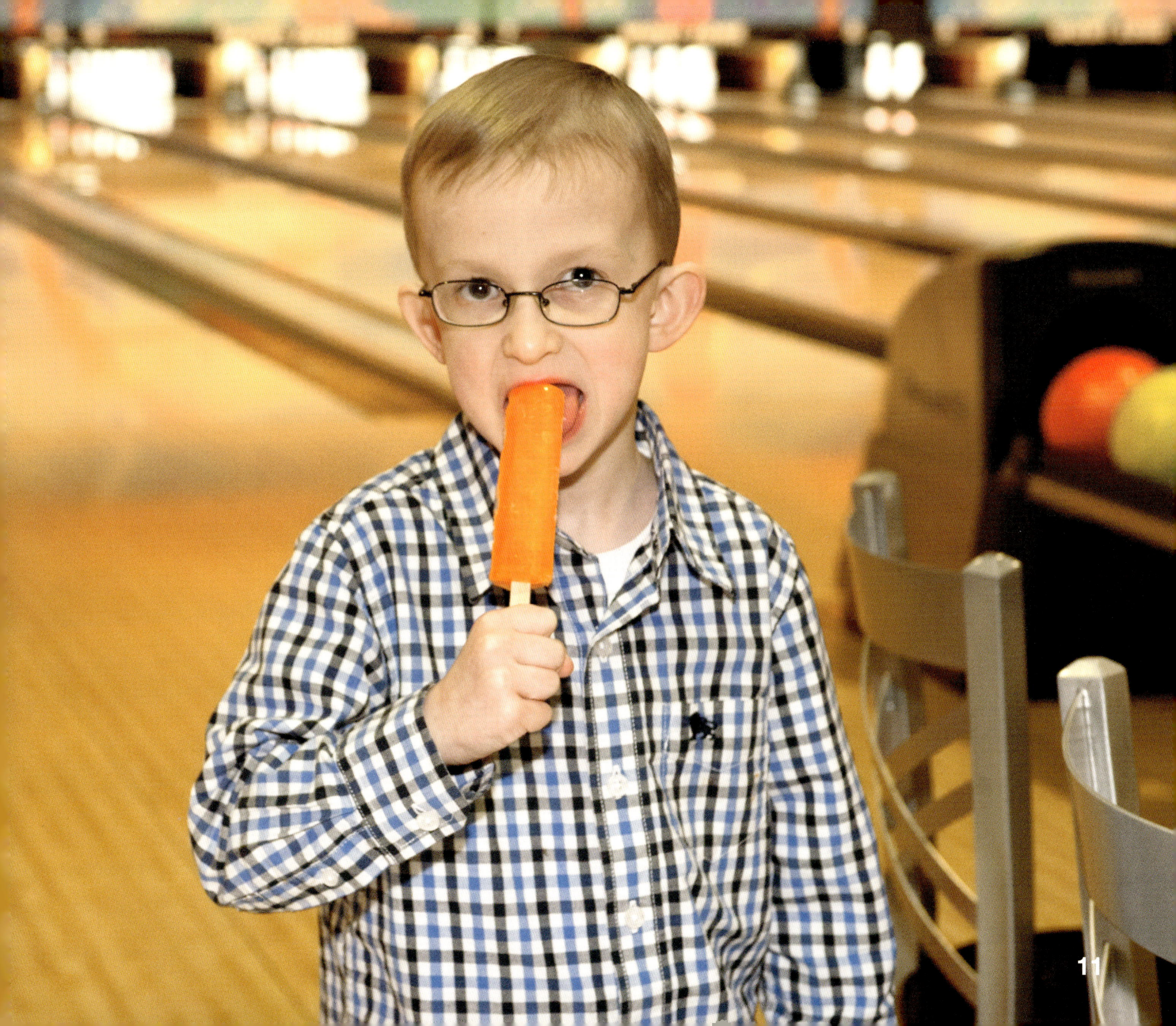

Eat Smart/ Come inteligentemente

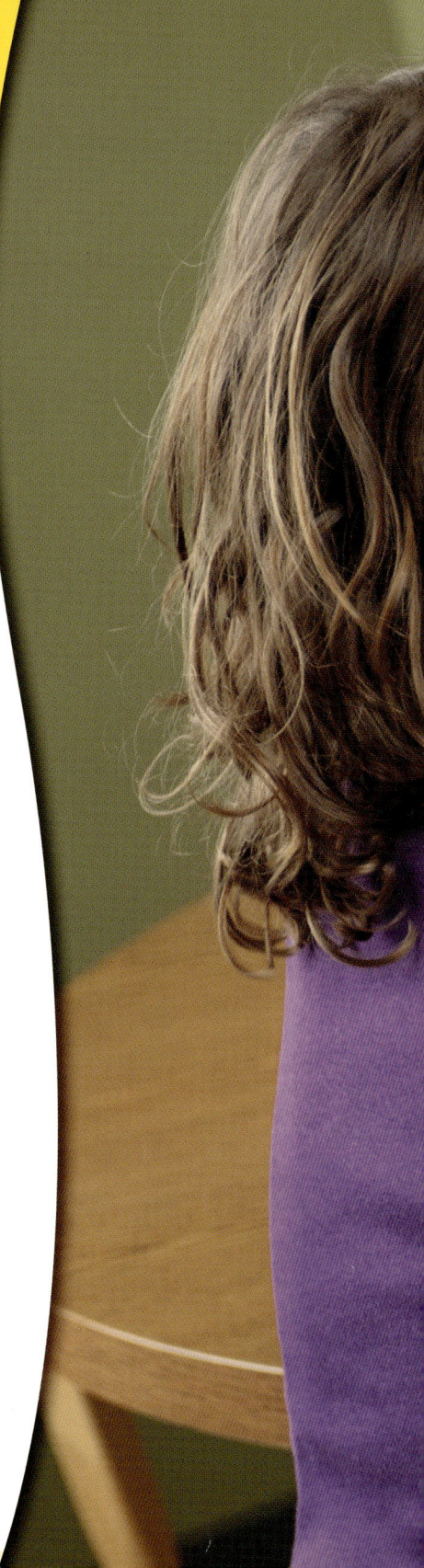

Enjoy sweets,
but eat fewer of them.
Share a small candy bar
with a friend.

Disfruta los dulces,
pero come menos de ellos.
Comparte una barrita de
chocolate con un amigo.

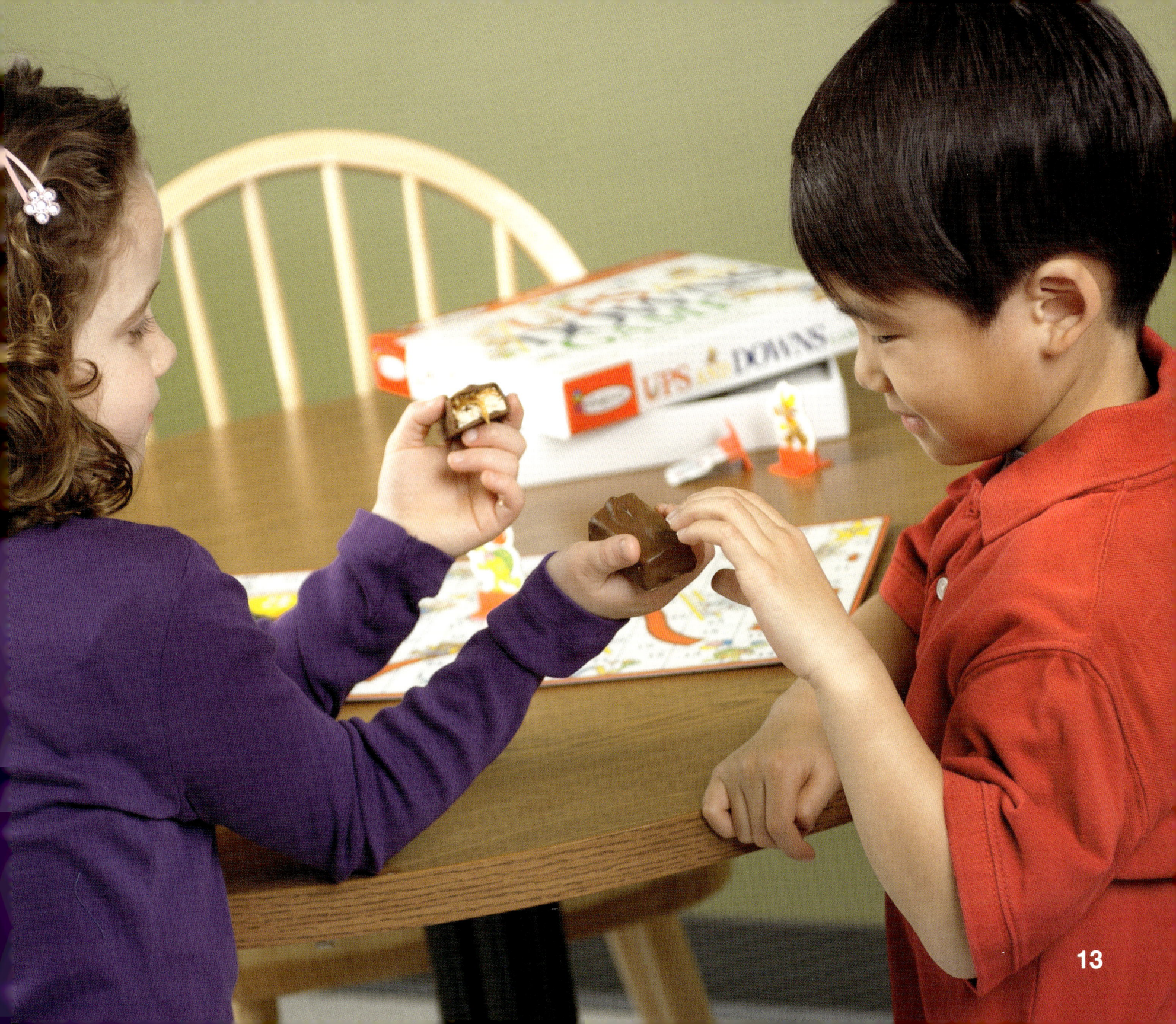

When it's time for a snack,

skip the chips.

Enjoy fresh fruit instead.

Cuando es hora de merendar,

no selecciones chips.

En su lugar, disfruta fruta fresca.

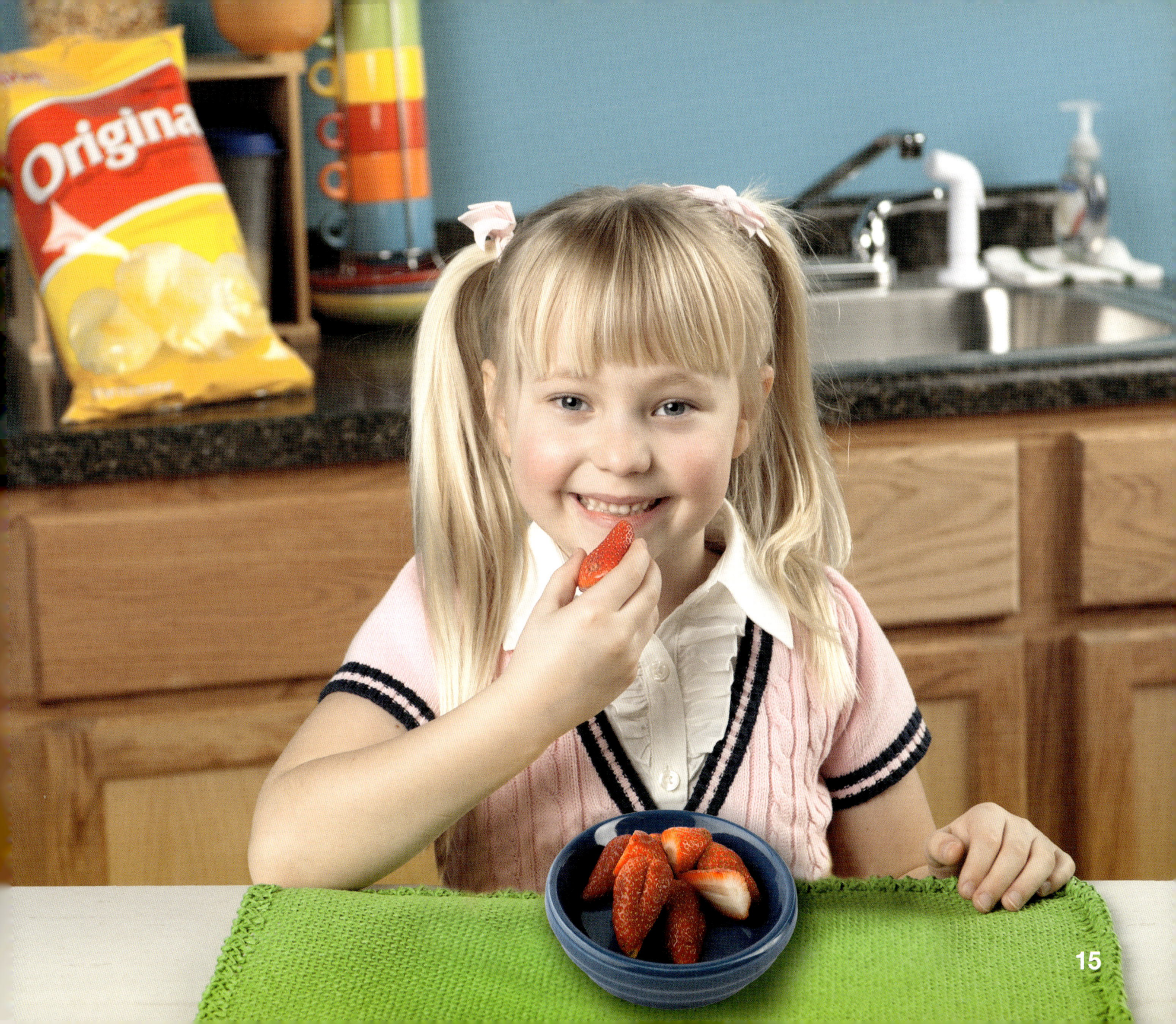

After dinner choose
a healthy dessert.
Enjoy a baked apple
or a frozen juice bar.

Después de la cena selecciona
un postre saludable.
Disfruta una manzana al horno
o helado de jugo de fruta.

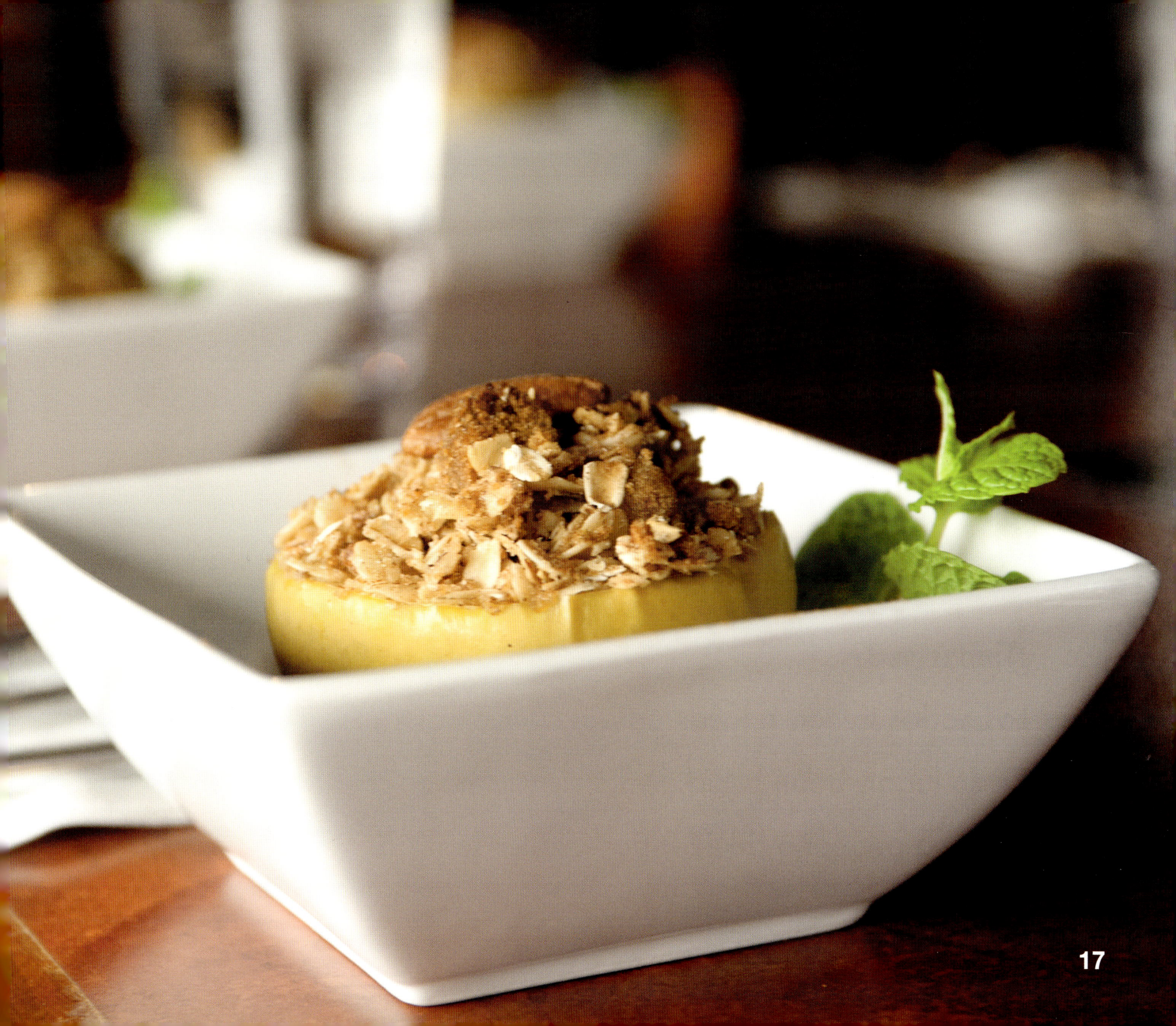

Are you thirsty?

Sodas have added sugar.

Drink water, skim milk, or a small glass of 100-percent juice instead.

¿Tienes sed?

Las sodas tienen azúcar agregada.

En su lugar, bebe agua, leche descremada o un vaso pequeño de 100 por ciento de jugo.

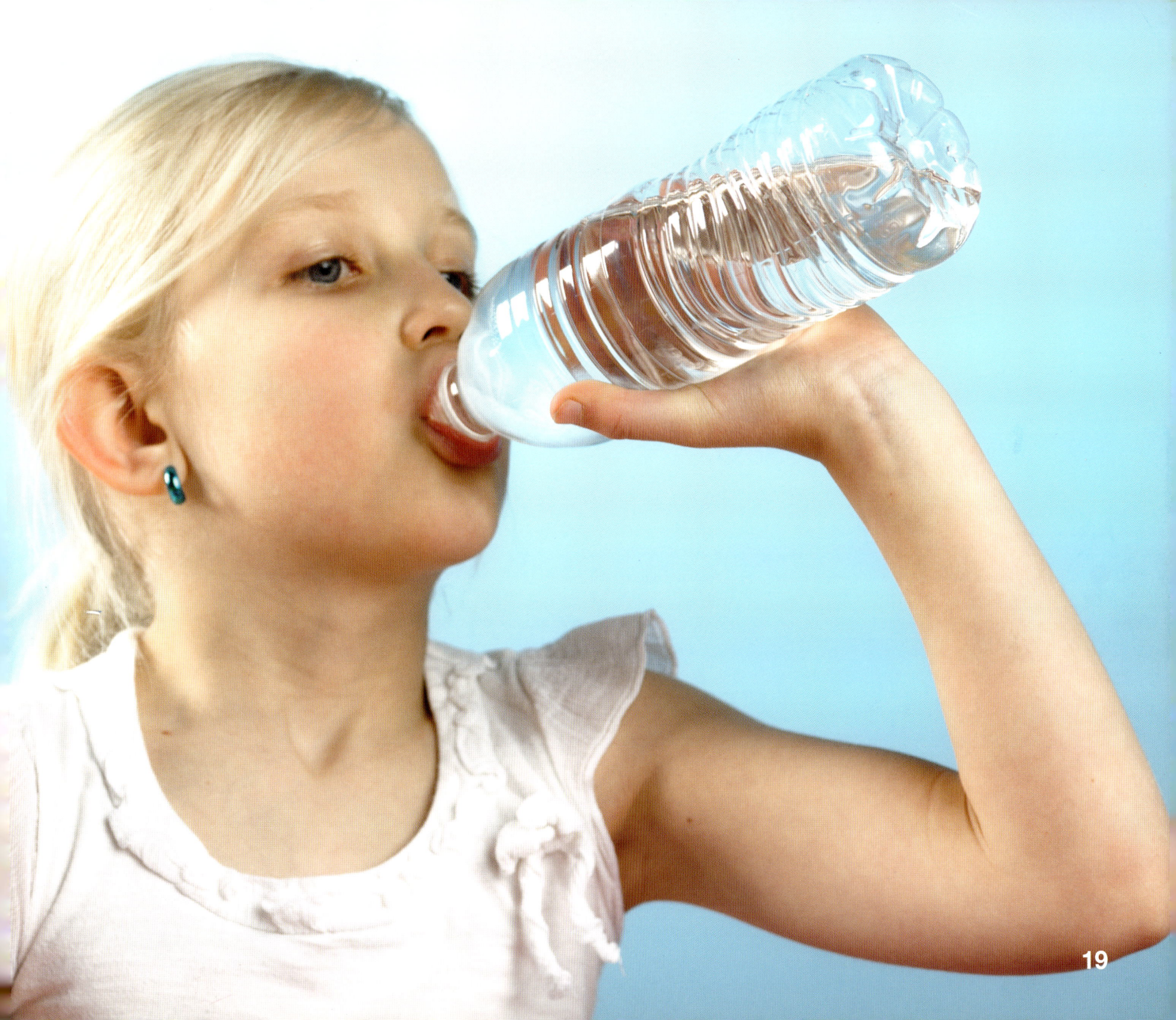

Making Healthy Choices

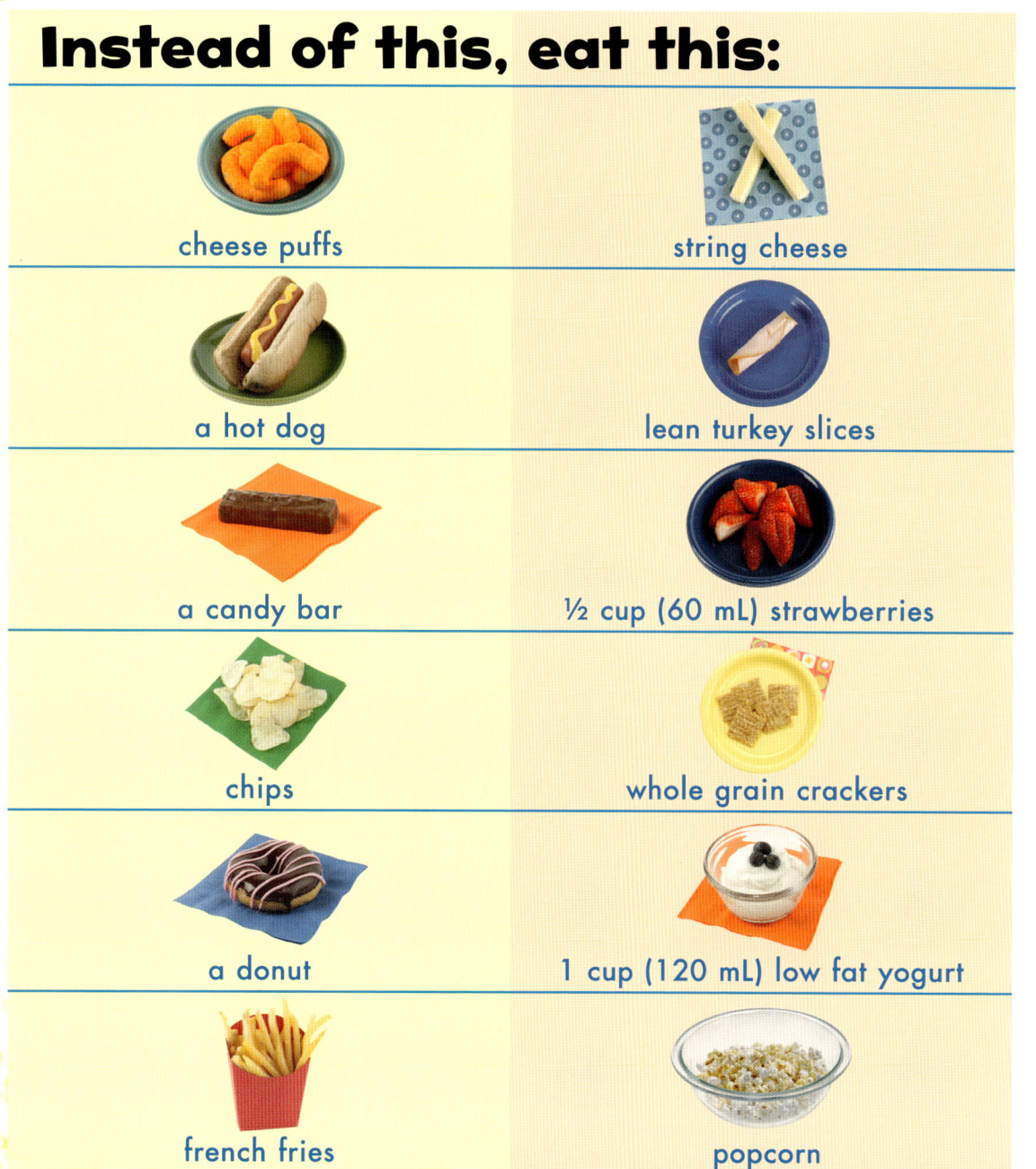

Instead of this, eat this:

cheese puffs	string cheese
a hot dog	lean turkey slices
a candy bar	½ cup (60 mL) strawberries
chips	whole grain crackers
a donut	1 cup (120 mL) low fat yogurt
french fries	popcorn

Cómo hacer selecciones saludables

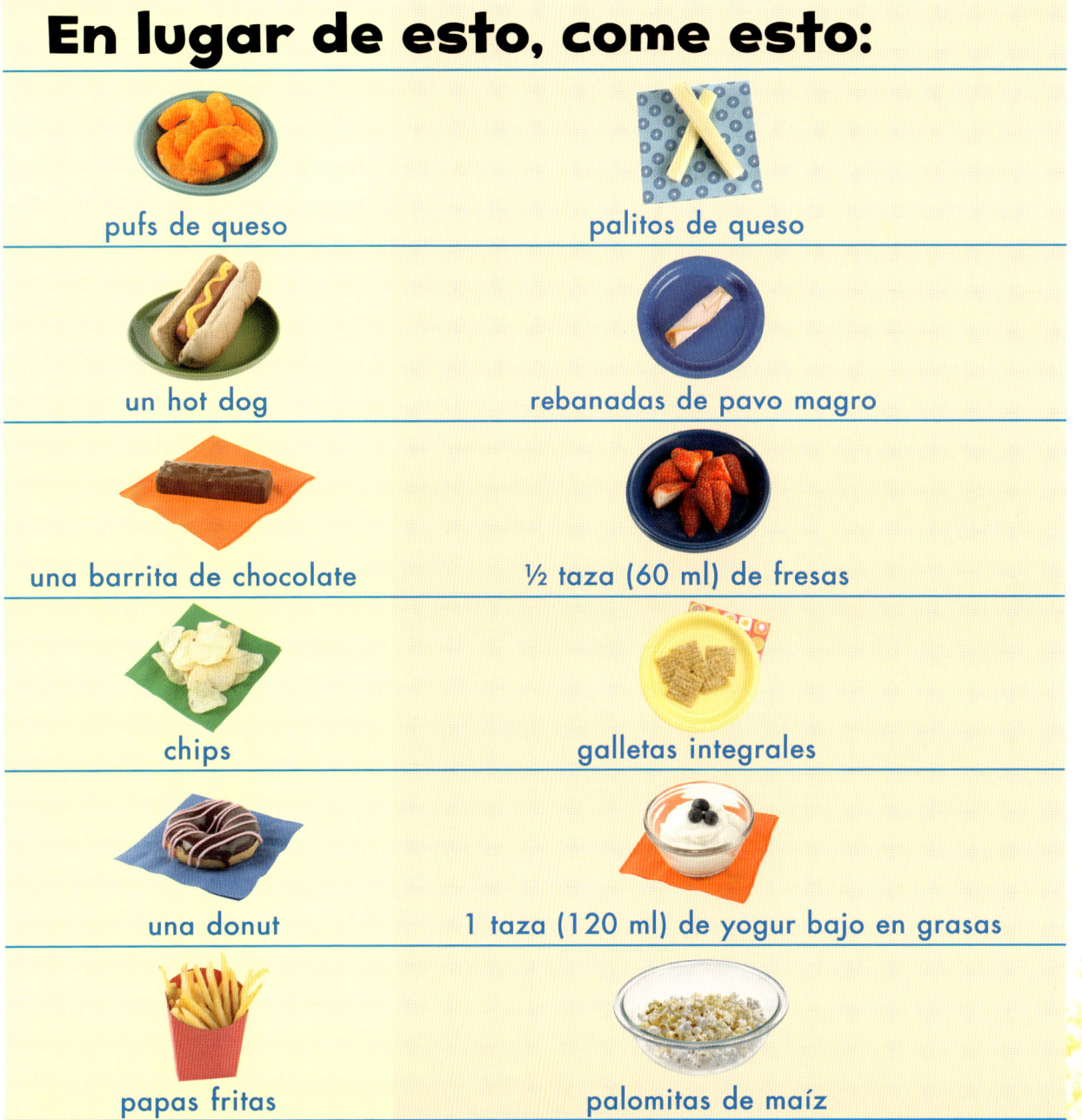

En lugar de esto, come esto:

pufs de queso	palitos de queso
un hot dog	rebanadas de pavo magro
una barrita de chocolate	½ taza (60 ml) de fresas
chips	galletas integrales
una donut	1 taza (120 ml) de yogur bajo en grasas
papas fritas	palomitas de maíz

Glossary

added sugar—any kind of sugar added to a food

MyPlate—a food plan that reminds people to eat healthful food and be active; MyPlate was created by the U.S. Department of Agriculture

nutrient—something that people need to eat to stay healthy and strong; vitamins and minerals are nutrients

snack—a small amount of food people eat between meals

solid fat—a kind of fat that is solid at room temperature; solid fat is also called saturated fat

sugar—a sweet substance that comes from plants

Internet Sites

FactHound offers a safe, fun way to find Internet sites related to this book. All of the sites on FactHound have been researched by our staff.

Here's all you do:

Visit www.facthound.com

Type in this code: 9781620659465

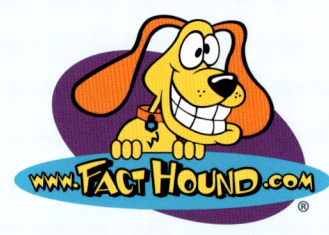

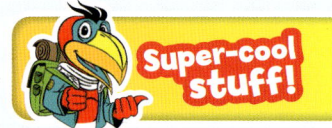

Check out projects, games and lots more at www.capstonekids.com

Glosario

el azúcar—una sustancia dulce que proviene de las plantas

el azúcar agregada—cualquier tipo de azúcar que se agrega a un alimento

la grasa sólida—un tipo de grasa que es sólida a temperatura ambiente; a la grasa sólida también se la llama grasa saturada

la merienda—una pequeña cantidad de alimento que la gente come entre comidas

MiPlato—un plan de alimentos que hace recordar a la gente de comer alimentos saludables y de estar activos; MiPlato fue creado por el Departamento de Agricultura de EE.UU.

el nutriente—algo que la gente necesita comer para mantenerse saludable y fuerte; las vitaminas y los minerales son nutrientes

Sitios de Internet

FactHound brinda una forma segura y divertida de encontrar sitios de Internet relacionados con este libro. Todos los sitios en FactHound han sido investigados por nuestro personal.

Esto es todo lo que tienes que hacer:

Visita *www.facthound.com*

Ingresa este código: 9781620659465

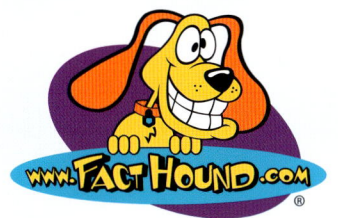

¡Algo súper divertido! Hay proyectos, juegos y mucho más en www.capstonekids.com

Index

desserts, 16
drinks, 18
fats, 4, 8, 10
limiting, 4, 10, 12

MyPlate, 4
nutrients, 6, 8
sugars, 4, 6, 10, 18
treats, 10

Índice

azúcares, 4, 6, 10, 18
bebidas, 18
golosinas, 10
grasas, 4, 8, 10

limitar, 4, 10, 12
MiPlato, 4
nutrientes, 6, 8
postres, 16